CLEA

The Therapeutic Medical Guide To
Heal Diseases, Cleanse & Detoxify
The Body For Total Well Being

Dr. George Ken

Table of Contents

CHAPTER ONE

INTRODUCTION

The liver is that the body's natural detoxifier because it cleanses the body of poisons and produces bile to support healthy digestion. A healthy liver can detoxify almost everything that an individual encounters. The liver is on the proper side of the body, slightly below the skeletal structure, when the liver is diseased; the body cannot filter toxic substances as efficiently. this will cause a good range of symptoms, including:

*   itching

*   yellow   jaundiced   skin

* swelling
* blood vessel problems
* gallstones
* fatigue
* nausea
* diarrhea

CHAPTER TWO

IMPORTANT FACTS YOU SHOULD KNOW

A detox is actually the method of removing toxins from the body; therefore the initiative is to scale back your consumption of refined sugars, tobacco, alcohol and excessive coffee. Then by incorporating a variety of super-foods to your diet, you'll naturally cleanse and protect this hard-working organ.
A healthy liver naturally cleanses itself. An unhealthy liver won't recover with a liver cleanse. an individual with disease needs

proper medical treatment and should require lifestyle or dietary changes. However, exposure to chemicals can damage the liver. For instance, drinking alcohol may be a well-known thanks to ruin liver function over time. In most cases, a liver detox involves one or more of the following:

a. taking supplements designed to flush toxins out of the liver

b. eating a liver-friendly diet

c. avoiding certain foods

d. going on a juice fast

e. cleansing the colon and gut through the utilization of enemas

While liver failure may be a

serious ill health , there's no evidence that dangerous toxins accumulate in otherwise healthy livers without specific exposure to large amounts of those chemicals.

FOODS THAT NATURALLY CLEANSE THE LIVER

*   Tea

Tea is widely considered to be beneficial for health; it's going to have benefits for the liver. Drinking 5 to 10 cups of tea each day was related to improved blood markers of liver health. This might be right down to a compound known to help liver function named catechin. Tea is packed filled with this plant antioxidant. Just be mindful of tea extract because it can have a negative effect.

* Cruciferous Vegetables this includes, but isn't limited to, broccoli, cauliflower, Brussels sprouts, cabbage and kale. These vegetables are a serious source of glutathione, which triggers the toxin cleansing enzymes of the liver. Eating cruciferous vegetables will increase production of glucosinolate in your system, which helps flush out carcinogens and other toxins.

* Turmeric

additionally to its use as a spice and pigment, turmeric has been utilized in India for medicinal purposes for hundreds of years. Curcumin is that the active ingredient in turmeric, and its powerful biological properties. This spice helps the enzymes that flush out toxins and contains antioxidants that repair liver cells. It also assists the liver in detoxing metals, while boosting bile production.

*   Citrus

While also providing an enormous hit of vitamin C, citrus fruits stimulate the liver and aid the synthesizing of toxic materials into substances which will be absorbed by water. Grapefruit is especially beneficial because it contains two primary antioxidants: naringin and naringenin. These may help protect the liver from injury by reducing inflammation and protecting the liver cells.

*   Beetroot

Beets also contain vitamin C and a healthy dose of fiber which are both natural cleansers for the gastrointestinal system . But more impressively, beets assist with increasing oxygen by cleansing the blood, and may break down toxic wastes to assist them be excreted quicker. They stimulate bile flow

and boost enzymatic activity.
* Garlic

Garlic is loaded with sulphur, which activates liver enzymes that help your body flush out toxins. Garlic also holds high amounts of selenium. Selenium is an important micronutrient that has been shown to assist boosts the natural antioxidant enzyme levels in our livers. Supplementing with selenium gives our livers even more ammunition within the fight against the damage caused by oxidative stress.
* Walnuts

Walnuts are an honest source of glutathione, omega-3 fatty acids, and therefore the aminoalkanoic acid arginine, which supports normal liver cleansing actions, especially when detoxifying ammonia.

* Olive Oil although it's a fat, vegetable oil is taken into account a healthy fat. Cold-pressed organic oils like olive, hemp, and flaxseed offer great support for the liver, providing the body with a liquid base which will suck up harmful toxins within the body. It's also been shown to decrease the amount of fat within the liver.

CHAPTER THREE

WHAT YOU NEED TO KNOW

Liver cleanses also pose some health   risks:

* Liver cleansing diets might not offer balanced nutrition: A liver cleansing diet might not contain all nutrients that an individual requires. Over time, this will cause deficiencies or malnutrition, particularly in children, pregnant women, and other people with diabetes and other medical conditions.

* Enemas are often dangerous: Enemas can cause life-threatening damage to the intestines when not

administered   correctly.

* Liver cleanses cannot replace medical treatment: When an individual uses a liver cleanse in situ of medical treatment, serious underlying medical issues can go untreated.

In fact, very low-calorie diets can slow the body's metabolism. This is often because the body adjusts to the low nutrient intake by absorbing nutrients more slowly. Some diets enhance liver health require people to consume few calories for several days. This will end in temporary weight loss. Much of the load loss, however, is water weight, which can return once an individual begins to eat normally again.

WAYS YOU CAN ENHANCE YOUR LIVER HEALTH

Some simple strategies which will reduce the danger of disease and help the liver rid the body of poisons include:
* Limiting alcohol intake: Excessive alcohol consumption may be a risk factor for disease. People with an addiction to alcohol should consider treatment.
* Avoiding unnecessary over the counter medications: Never exceed the recommended dose,

particularly of medicine like acetaminophen which will harm the liver. Don't mix alcohol and over the counter drugs.
* Choosing reputable tattoo and piercing salons: Choose a salon that sterilizes their equipment. Unsafe body modifications can transmit hepatitis C.
* Getting vaccinated: an individual should get vaccinated for hepatitis A and B, and confirm they get appropriate vaccinations before traveling overseas.
* Practicing safe sex: this will reduce the danger of transmitting conditions that affect the liver. People should also get tested

regularly for sexually transmitted infections.

* Avoiding potentially dangerous chemicals: When painting or using pesticides wear a mask and make sure the area is well ventilated.

* Drinking many water.

*Rinsing fruit and vegetables: this will help ensure they're freed from pesticides.

CHAPTER FOUR

WHAT TO EAT

a. Garlic: Garlic contains selenium, a mineral that helps to detoxify the liver. It also has the power to activate liver enzymes which will help your body naturally flush out toxins.
b. Citrus Fruits: Fruits like grapefruit, oranges, limes and lemons all boost the liver's cleansing ability. Even consumed in small amounts citrus fruits help the liver to supply the detoxifying enzymes that flush out pollutants.
* Vegetables: Cruciferous

vegetables like broccoli and cauliflower contain glucosinolate, which helps the liver to supply detoxifying enzymes. They also contain sulfur compounds that aid with liver health. Leafy vegetables are high in chlorophyll, which leaches toxins out of the blood stream. They will neutralize heavy metals to guard the liver.

* Turmeric: This herb works wonders for the liver it helps the enzymes that flush out toxins and contains antioxidants that repair liver cells. It also assists the liver in detoxing metals, while boosting bile production.

* Walnuts: Walnuts are high

within the aminoalkanoic acid arginine and assist the liver in detoxifying ammonia. They're high in glutathione and omega-3 fatty acids, which all provide support to natural liver cleansing.
* Beets: Beets assist with increasing oxygen by cleansing the blood, and may break down toxic wastes to assist them be excreted quicker. They stimulate bile flow and boost enzymatic activity. Beets also contain fiber and vitamin C, which both are natural cleansers for the gastrointestinal system.
* Carrots: Carrots are very high in plant-flavonoids and beta-carotene, which stimulates and

supports liver function overall. They also contain vitamin A, which prevents disease.
* Green Tea: If you're thirsty from all the liver-benefiting foods, try some tea . This beverage contains catechins, plant-based antioxidants known to enhance liver function. Take care to stay to tea and not tea extract, which may potentially negatively impact liver health.
* Apples: Apples contain high levels of pectin, a chemical that helps the body cleanse and release toxins from the alimentary canal. With fewer toxins within the alimentary canal, the liver can

better manage its toxin load, having the ability to rose cleanse the remainder of the body. *Avocado: Avocados are basically a superfood. Additionally to cleansing your arteries, they assist the body naturally produce glutathione, the compound that helps the liver rid itself of poisons. * The liver is that the organ that filters, processes and breaks down what passes through your body. It's liable for filtering your blood and helping it to clot, breaking down any chemicals, alcohol and medicines you're taking in while producing glucose and bile, two important substances you would like to remain healthy. * When the liver becomes overwhelmed with toxins and pollutants, its natural working cycle slows down. Besides alcohol, drugs and other taxing chemicals, we tend to overload our livers with processed and fried foods, especially when consumed in large quantities.

THE END

Made in the USA
Monee, IL
27 June 2021

72411431R00015